This book is dedicated to my wonderful wife, Arlene, for being my partner in life. You have helped me with every aspect of this book, especially giving me the love and support I needed to make it a reality.

To our sons, Don & Joel, and daughter Laurie, along with son-in-law, Norman Regal: Each of them is a fitness buff in their own special way.

And to you the reader, your body and mind are what you've been given at birth. Build on your base and treat them with care.

You are the master of your own destiny.

Train hard, eat well, and live your life in

Good health and happiness.

# Introduction

Welcome to Fitness - First & Forever. I hope you find this book as interesting and informative as it was for me to compose and publish it. It is different from most of the material that you've read on exercise in that the approach is from a different background. Exercising the body via workouts affects all structures of the human body and is the best 'medicine' one can take for positive results and with few negative side effects.

I started working out as a youngster and since then I have been exercising and studying fitness, on and off, as time would allow. Since my retirement as a dentist, the subject of fitness has filled most of my time. As a general dentist I was always concerned about my patient's oral health. Before long into retirement I became interested in becoming a personal trainer. So a new profession and goal was to be established for my future. Studying for the test to become a certified personal trainer was like reviewing some the subjects I had in dental school. What fun! In this case rather than treating patients, I would work with clients in a gym!

Medical doctors and dentists spend the first 2 years of professional school learning essentially the same subject matter. The basic physical life of a human is reflected in studying biochemistry, histology, microbiology, anatomy, physiology, pathology, patient care, diagnosis, biomaterials, treatment of disease, medications and healing. In addition, the medical doctor and dentist see patients in pain, nervous about their condition and concerned about their choice of treatments.

In training others as a personal trainer, all of the above subjects aided in prescribing a course for a workout routine. Client's have to be evaluated as to their health, medications they take, if any, their time allotments for working out, and any physical impairments they may have. Consultations with their doctors by the trainer may be necessary.

Besides seeing clients in a gym or at their home, their progress in firming their body, losing fat, building muscle and strength, often leads to their desire to learn more about fitness and exercise. Contacting clients via their e-mail address, providing them with interesting matters on exercising, sleep, diet, and has always perked their motivation.

Fitness involves 4 basic pillars that one must follow to get the maximum benefit for the time and practice it requires by the trainee. They are (1) an exercise program, (2) follow a nutritious diet, (3) get adequate sleep, (4) rest - allow enough time for your muscles to rebuild after high intensity exercising.

# Table of Contents

Dedication

Introduction

**Part One: Matters Concerning Exercise**

Who Are You?

Fitness Explained

Fitness Sources of Information

To Succeed in Your Fitness Program You Need to Motivate Yourself

Exercise – Some Facts and Myths

Movement vs. Exercise

What Happens When You Exercise?

Learn "Muscle Talk"

Exercising – No Gym

How to Choose a Personal Trainer

Strength Training

Interval Training

Breathing While Exercising

The Interrelated Components of Fitness

Training for Beginners

Training for Beginners – Part 2

Strength Training for Seniors

Strength Training for Seniors – A Research Report

Sarcopenia


Muscular Fitness vs. Body Weight

The Couch Potato

# Part 2:  Your Diet

Your Diet – The Simple Approach

Diet & Facts You Should know

Nutrition – A Recommended Diet

The Mediterranean Diet

The Mediterranean Diet; a Summary of Research Studies

Sugar & Spice Makes Nothing Nice

# Part 3:  Sleep

What Happens During Sleep

The What and Why of a "Sleep Study"

Sleep Apnea

Sleeping Positions Can Affect Sleep

## Part 4:  Hormones

Exercise; How it Affects your Hormones

Hormones and Weight Control

Factors Affecting Metabolic Demands

## References

# Who Are You?

What a bizarre question to ask someone and how many answers are there to this inquiry? You may be one thing to your spouse, something else to your boss or friend but who are you, meaning YOU, personally. The answer, here at least, may influence your life and what to expect of yourself.

Being a homo sapien, you are a member of the animal group, and probably one of the most complex entities in the universe. You could fill a book on who you are, why and how you function, what to expect of yourself, and how you can be "all that you could be" without becoming a U.S. Marine!

Our human family originated about 200,000 years ago in the Middle Paleolithic period in southern Africa. Whether produced by a super-natural being, or developed as part of an evolutionary process, we have component parts that help us dictate what we do, and how we do it.

Let's begin at birth and look at what we are, anatomically, biologically, and even under the microscope. It's been estimated that a human is made of approximately 37 + trillion (that's spelled with a "T") cells. We have approximately 206 bones, 630 muscles, 50 hormones and 243 joints. Oh, we also have ligaments, tendons, skin, fat, internal organs, and umpteen million other components. We have the most developed brain of all the animals in our group, and with a central nervous system (CNS). The CNS is composed of 24 cranial nerves (12 pairs) and 64 spinal nerves (32 pairs). It also has over a billion branches.  Each of our cells is a small chemical factory that needs nutrition to produce what we need to nourish our body.

So what's this have to do with fitness you ask?  If you want to function in health and live a vibrant life, you, Mr. CEO, have been installed in your corporation whether you like it or not.  You have a lot to learn about yourself and don't rely on your doctor because he is, essentially, a facilitator. He may help you with your pains, high blood pressure, and osteoporosis, but he cannot do your healing for you. That's up to you and how well you control your corporation, from birth to the present time.

As you view the components of your body, you realize that the bones give shape and structure to our bodies, the ligaments attach bones to bones and tendons attach muscles to bones and joints.  The purpose and instruction our creator has given us is to use what we have, maintain our health and tend to our needs as humans.  We are a miraculous creation that thinks, understands, moves and heals itself.  We are not machines that go in for service every 5000 miles.  How about daily?

# Fitness Explained

Wikipedia's definition of Fitness is as follows:
"**Physical fitness** is a general state of <u>health</u> and well being or specifically the ability to perform aspects of <u>sports</u> or occupations. Physical fitness is generally achieved through correct <u>nutrition</u>, <u>exercise</u>, <u>hygiene</u> and rest. It is a set of attributes or characteristics that people have or achieve that relates to the ability to perform physical activity." This field is in a constantly changing mode, both in the information developed by research and in the practice of all those fields related to fitness. Short form – it's what you should know and incorporate in your daily "to do's" if your health and well being have meaning to you.

Here are some of the topics we see and hear daily. Do this and that to lose weight, eat low fat/high fat foods, more lower calorie foods, you need more vitamins A-Z, drink 10 glasses of water, blah,blah, blah. How do you know what to believe? A suggestion: Eat fresh vegetables, fruits, meat, fish, chicken, turkey, and watch your diet to get enough fiber. When you get thirsty, trust your senses to tell you when to drink liquids. Lean to read food labels and check to keep all forms of sugar low. Sugar is an irritant to the body and a lot of it is a no-no. The sugar (fructose) in fruit should suffice and stay away from man-made pastry, pies, cookies, and candies.

Please realize that when claims are made in most matters of life, including fitness, the research to verify the safety and benefits of various products arrives long after what is seen as advertisements on TV and in the news.

If you hear some news about a great product being advertised, contact the producer to give you the research done backing up the advertising of the company. Who did the research, who paid for the research, how many people were involved as test patients, was it done at a university, etc.?

Remember this and it's important – Exercise is the best medicine, with the fewest negative side effects, and you can do it at home or at a gym. The entire body responds positively and you'll have fewer chronic diseases, pain, obesity, etc., etc.

# Fitness Sources of Information

As your interest in fitness increases, as it probably will, I suggest you consider the sources listed below for obtaining answers to the questions you may have. You may read different blogs, newspapers, or watch something on the TV about how to lose 25 lbs. of fat in 3 weeks. Maybe it's how to get all the benefits of exercising in 12 minutes a week. Don't get confused and take the wrong source of information!

Search the web and you can find differing views on most subjects, so it's necessary that you don't get led astray and just give up on your exercise program. Most of what you read can come from actual research but the mavens on exercise can differ as to their interpretation of the facts.

If common sense doesn't answer your questions, you can contact the follow websites:

1. Journal of Strength and Conditioning; https://www.google.com/?gws_rd=ssl#q=journal+of+strength+and+conditioning
2. Journal of Applied Physiology, Nutrition and Metabolism; http://www.nrcresearchpress.com/doi/abs/10.1139/H07-123#.VC7hGdzF9LM
3. Journal of Clinical Endocrinology and Metabolism;

http://en.wikipedia.org/wiki/The_Journal_of_Cli
nical_Endocrinology_and_Metabolism
4. American Journal of Clinical Nutrition;
http://ajcn.nutrition.org/
5. International Journal of Obesity and Related
Metabolic Disorders;
http://www.ncbi.nlm.nih.gov/nlmcatalog?term=I
nternational+journal+of+obesity+and+related+
metabolic+disorders%5BTitle%5D
6. National Institutes of Health Office of Dietary
Supplements; http://ods.od.nih.gov/
7. Proceedings of the Nutrition Society;
http://www.nutritionsociety.org/publications/nutr
ition-society-journals/proceedings-of-the-
nutrition-society

Note: In reading some of the more technical articles, go to the 'Conclusion' and see the author's condensation of his (their) research. This will save you time, and reduce the frustration in trying to understand what really matters.

Other reliable sources on the treatment of diseases, diets, supplements and medical problems in general, consider the Mayo Clinic; www.mayoclinic.org.

and/or the Cleveland Clinic; https://www.google.com/?gws_rd=ssl#q=clevel and+clinic

# To Succeed in Your Fitness Program You need to Motivate Yourself

### 1. Set your goals.
With paper in hand, write down reasonable goals to follow and date each goal in the future.  Example: Lose 10 lbs by (date); reduce waste measurement by 1 inch by (date).

### 2. This is your time - no interruptions.
Conversations are okay if kept to a minimum, but remember why you came to the gym in the first place! Plan your workouts as time allows, but try to save 30-60 minutes for yourself.  If you're really serious about fitness, leave the cell phone in the locker while you are in the gym. Concentrate on what you're doing.  It's not the time that counts but rather what you do with it.

### 3.  Have fun during your workout.
No matter what form of exercise you do, what do you like to do for the long run? Perhaps you may consider one type of exercising along with another.  Example: Jog three times a week and strength train for three alternate days.  Variety improves the attitude and interest in exercising.

## 4.  Consistency is the name of the game.
Plan your routine for long term practice.  If you stop or interrupt your fitness plan, how will you make up for the time you lost doing other things?

## 5. Intensity training.
After a period of conditioning you should start increasing the work load you place on yourself to reach a higher level of development.  Let's say you are a beginner, deconditioned and somewhat of a couch potato.  If you are basically in good health and get checkups by your medical doctor as required, what was a little difficult to do as a beginner became easier as you progressed in your fitness routine. All forms of physical exercise require an increasing intensity to progress.  If you do the same type of exercise without pushing yourself, you remain in a static physical condition.  If you want to reach your goals, increased energy and effort is required.

## 6. Attitude.
Like everything we do in life, our attitude influences our happiness (or lack of it), smile, stress, work, workouts, and many other conditions. Strive to have a positive attitude.  If something bothers you, and you have no control over its outcome, practice ignoring it. Negative attitudes case stress without a payoff!

## 7. Keep an open mind and fill it with good information.
If you plan a fitness routine considers a variety of different exercises, working on the whole body and not only a selected area (abs as an example).  Look at fitness and exercise books, talk to trainers, and look in the mirror to see how you are progressing.

Check for flabby areas, pot bellies, weak muscles, poor balance.  Obtain and keep copies of your medical records and read them!  Check your blood counts and see if they are within normal limits.  Before visiting your doctor, make a list of questions you would like him to answer.  Bring in an updated list and amounts of all medications you take.

## 8. Year in - year out.
Please remember that you, and only you, live in your body.  Keep it healthy by good nutrition, exercise, adequate rest and sleep and enjoyment in each and every day.  It will reduce your aches and pains, chronic disease, and medical bills.  Your fitness routine should be planned for day to day and year to year practice.  Enroll in your "college of fitness".

# Exercise - Some Facts & Myths

In 1968 Kenneth Cooper, MD wrote a book called Aerobics and it has been updated since then. Dr. Cooper's book was very popular and had a lot of good information that could be used in an exercise program. He has been credited with popularizing aerobic exercising and some of the examples he referred to in his book are jogging, running, sprinting, using treadmill, step machines, elliptical trainers, and the list goes on and on. Unfortunately, exercise as taught by trainers, in gym, at high schools, and many other places, are using the word "aerobics", incorrectly. All members of the animal kingdom live aerobically, meaning they need oxygen to live. For a human to exercise anaerobically (without oxygen) is nonsense. An animal without oxygen is a corpse or on the way to becoming one. Note: ALL EXERCISE IS AEROBIC and to refer to weight lifting, hill climbing, isometrics; yoga or any movement at all as anaerobic is not realistic and should be recognized accordingly.

Perhaps the concept of aerobics/anaerobic developed by how energy is produced. The body produces energy in a complex system called the tricarboxylic acid cycle or Krebs's Cycle.  The cycle is a series of reactions that occur in specialize organelles called mitochondria. The energy component, ATP (Adenosine Tri-Phosphate), is produced in this cycle along with some other products such as lactic acid, oxygen, amino acids, fatty acids, and glucose.  The initial ATP and the lactic acid are produced anaerobically but the total body does not function without oxygen. Try to think of the human energy systems as continuous, just like a circle and the result of the energy system is, yep, you guessed it, the production of ENERGY!

So to sum it all up let's call running, jugging, sprinting, elliptical training and other machines designed to speed up the heart, "cardio training" and not aerobics.  Weight or strength training, yoga, Pilate's, are all aerobic.  To sum up, everything a human does is aerobic.  To those that don't believe this statement try doing any form of exercise with duct tape covering your nose and mouth!

# Movement vs. Exercise

For anyone that exercises or teaches exercise either as a trainer in a gym or as an instructor in a school, one has to know the difference between movement and exercise. Unfortunately, too many who "exercise" do movements and think they are benefiting from it.

It is not easy to find a definition of exercise and it usually is defined by its goals; provide increasing strength, endurance, flexibility, etc. Exercise is really movement of one's whole body (as in running or swimming) or parts of the body (as in a bicep curl or as in a deep knee bend). The difference between movement and exercise is the extent of exertion and intensity that is involved. Also exercise is performed with critical care in execution and form. Movement is much less concerned about form, time, intensity, and body changes over a period of time.

Exercise is movement - plus. It involves the coordination of nerves, muscles, bones, joints, resistance, time, endurance, intensity and effort. It starts with low effort and progresses to increased intensity and fatigue of the muscles being utilized.

Exercise can be characterized by an increase in breathing rate, heart rate, perspiration, energy expenditure (calories), and increased intensity of movement to the extent of failure to perform more repetitions.  There are also internal changes within the body involving the nervous system, hormonal changes, chemical changes from the time food is eaten and all the way through the digestive track.  To get an idea of what's involved go to your browser, (Google search, Bing,) and post: Krebs's cycle with equations.  It will blow your mind! Krebs's cycle illustrates how energy is produced so that you can move, exercise, go shopping or go fishing.

An example is a walk around the block.  It is definitely movement of the total body but not necessarily to the extent of it being an exercise.  Realize that productive exercise is intensified movement characterized by what is mentioned above.

A beginner should learn what and how to do the movements to make them into an exercising procedure.  Like most everything else in life that is of value, one has to pay the price to advance to a goal.  In a workout, the results you get are totally dependent and proportional to the amount of effort you expend, but more about that in an upcoming posting.

How do you know if you are exercising enough or too much?  How do you feel when your workout period is over? How about the next day? If you feel like you put in a good effort, with increasing intensity, and follow through each exercise to fatigue and your last repetition is really your last repetition that you can possible do, you've done enough!  If you are an experienced trainee, you can continue on with your exercise by doing a set or two using lighter weights.

The reason for increasing the intensity and work load is to recruit more and more of the muscle fibers. They are the structures in the muscles that contract and expand. The next day you probably will feel stiff, have some muscle tenderness, may not be quit as limber, and may be sensitive to pressure on some spots around your body. Good for you! You did it right the last time you worked out. Give yourself a day's rest or work on different set of muscles in you exercise daily.

Too much exercise will reduce your progress and slow the attainment of your exercising goals. If you exercise properly, eat intelligently with the consumption of a well-rounded diet, and get enough sleep and rest, you shouldn't run into any trouble.

# What Happens When You Exercise?

There are times when you can take a very complicated subject like muscle physiology and metaphorically simplify it for "Dummies". No, this isn't meant to be a degrading of any one's intelligence, but rather to create a means to memorize any subject easier, longer, and more comprehensively. Let's get started.

An army is composed of soldiers and a muscle is made up of muscle fibers. These are the basic starting units within our discussion. Some of the soldiers drive tanks, other's are in the infantry and some man anti-aircraft canons (or guns). The soldiers are given specialized tasks. Muscle fibers are grouped together to form different muscle bundles that also do specialized work. Examples are the quadriceps that extends the leg, and the hamstrings flex the knee joint while extending the hip joint.

Exercise is basically "medicine" for the muscles, but causes the muscles to respond differently than you may imagine. Exercising does not build muscles; it causes a break-down process called catabolism. There is microscopic bleeding, tearing, and irritation of the muscle fibers. This process is magnified and enhanced during high intensity training (HIT). When you leave the gym the muscles are repaired by nutrition and rest, especially sleep. The results are found in muscles that are enlarged (hypertrophied) and increased in number (more muscle fibers are formed; hyperplasia). This process is a building stage called anabolism (as opposed to catabolism).

So if you want a strong army you need many soldier's that are trained, physically, to fight, endure, and "win the battle". With exercise, you want to recruit as many muscle fibers as possible, train them, with the result of having a stronger, healthier and firmer body. The human body is really a muscle machine designed to move.

There are specialized organelles, mostly in muscle, called mitochondria. They are responsible for developing energy to move the body, run, stretch, play tennis, etc. When people go on weight reducing diets, besides loosing fat, they also lose muscle tissue. It's essential to exercise when going on a diet, as it is all the time during your life in your body. If there is a sizable reduction in muscle substance, energy production is reduced, and can lead to a life of the "couch potato".

Kinesiology is the study of muscular movement and physiology. It is a subject major in many colleges and universities. There are many other benefits of exercising and books have been written of this subject. Please refer to the article on Strength Training in this book.

# Learn "Muscle Talk"

This is the basis of all exercise (arguably) and is not usually mentioned as something to learn. Too bad, as all trainees of any sport are involved with this "language". Listen up; The muscles have no brain cells, no hearing nerves, and the same goes for the smell, vision, speech and some of the other senses (up to 22 senses according to some scientists). They don't know the difference between 8 reps, 3 sets, or a Cobb salad! So if we want to develop our body to become strong, healthy, lean, and sexy, we have to understand ...........MUSCLE TALK!

If muscles don't talk, how can you understand what they want, what bothers them and what they can do? Let's say someone or some where you were led to believe that you should do a bicep curl for 10 reps and 3 sets. That's nice but it means nothing to the force that does the curl. The brain tells the muscles (via the nervous system) that you should pick up a dumbbell weighting 10 lbs and curl it 8 times. If you are strong enough to do it, you will, and maybe you can curl more than 10 lbs. How about 15 or 20 lbs? Sooner or later you won't be able to budge the added weight, even though your brain told you to execute the movement. What then? Instead of what then, consider what is the dominant force that is doing the exercise. The muscles told the brain to "Buzz off, we can't lift that amount of weight even for 1 rep" The muscles then prevail, right? So what this all means is that there is a final point in exercising that shows up when the muscles involved get progressively fatigued until failure of doing the curl. Whoopee! That point may be for 1, 5, or 15 reps or whatever. To read that you should use 10 lbs. for 8 reps is just a guess, by the trainee or trainer.

*Note: Doing exercising until failure is not something the beginner should practice. Learn how to do each exercise in good form for approximately 8-12 reps, and usually for 1 set. As your body responds to exercise wait for at least 1 month before increasing the intensity of the exercises performed. Also, it's advisable to have a trainer help you set up a program according to your condition, health and age.*

The description of exercise then becomes the progressive fatiguing of the muscles involved until failure of the movement, and it is done under supervision. The Supervisor then becomes the trainee's muscles.

# Exercising - No Gym

Not everyone can or wants to go to a gym for working out. If you are home, or away from home....not to worry! Can you lift a weight? How about a smart phone (cell phone)? You're stronger than you thought so now is the time to focus on exercising. Remember, it's the best medicine you can take, it's cheap, not very time consuming, and helps preserve good health.

If you can get out of bed, visit the toidy, and walk to your breakfast table without shortness of breath you have no excuses not to work out. If you are overweight, your first exercise is to push yourself away from your table after eating a smaller portion than you're used to. Also keep the portions no larger than your fist. You may search on the internet for nutrition, diet, and fitness information. If you are in really bad shape, consult with your doctor and see what he recommends relative to exercising and diet control.

There are certain principles you should follow if you plan to structure an exercise program without help from a trainer or knowledgeable person trained in exercising.
Rather than look at a book for pictures of how to perform any exercise, check out online videos for descriptions, before and after views on each exercise, and the author's comments. They are listed below and not necessarily in order of importance:

1.    Videos are available for your desktop, laptop, tablet, and/or smart cell phones that are much better than viewing photos or drawings in a book.

2.    Try to include the major muscle groups in any exercise program.  They are chest, back, abs, legs, arms and shoulders..

3.    Work out on core exercises, balance, stretching, and aerobics if you can.

4.    Don't expect exercise to lose weight.  Look to an intelligent diet you can follow and include exercising to maintain your muscles in good condition.  If you only diet and not exercise you can lose weight, including fat and muscle - not good, McGee! Save the muscles for later.  You'll need them!

Walking, jogging, and running outside or around a track are excellent examples of exercise.  You can do any of them with a friend or your dog.

Some sites you may want to visit for help in setting up an exercise routine are:

1.    Ace Fitness Programs with 25 exercises.

2.    The Huntington Post Crash Course of Exercising at Home.

3.    The No-equipment Workout You Can Do At Home (www.Oprah.com).

4.    Wiki - How to Exercise (has a very good description of various exercises).

# How to Choose a Personal Trainer

If you plan to use a personal trainer to help train you during your workouts you should prepare yourself as to the qualities you're looking for in your future "coach." What you're looking for is someone who makes you feel comfortable enough to accept their instruction and guidance. You want to tell them what you want to improve, what your goals are, and what health factors have to be considered, if any. Do you get short of breath, do you want to lose weight, how about firming your body, etc., etc.? Your trainer can help you achieve your goals and he/she should also be a motivator. Let's consider the following items:

Is the trainer an NCCA-accredited certification holder? The National Commission for Certifying Agencies (NCCA) has 26 years of experience accrediting many allied health professions such as nurses, dietitians, athletic trainers and occupational therapists. You can check on the trainer's credential's by visiting www.noca.org and then clink on the NCCA link. Some of the more popular and established accredited organizations include The American Council on Exercise (ACE), the National Academy of Sports Medicine (NASM), and the National Strength and Conditioning Association (NSCA). Also how long has he been actively training clients?

Discuss with the trainer his/her work experience and area of specialization. Is the trainer able to consult with your doctor if you have any medical problems that he should be aware of?

Does the trainer have any letters of recommendation from former clients?  Would he mind if you contacted any of them on the phone?  How about previous employers that he has worked for as a certified personal trainer?

Does he carry a professional liability insurance policy?  Does the gym he works for carry liability insurance?

Does the trainer seem to have patience and interest in what the two of you are discussing? If he doesn't "mesh" with your personality, don't get involved and look for another trainer that you think will fill you requirements.........with a smile on his face!

Does the trainer exhibit professionalism?  Try and watch how he trains someone else
before deciding on agreeing to become his client.
 Does he look interested in his client or just count reps?  Does he teach or spend time on other matters relating to fitness?
Does he use your time to talk on his cell phone to someone else?

What is his background in his area of expertise?
 Does he prefer younger clients?  How about seniors?
 Try to find someone who feels comfortable and experienced in your age group of clients.

If you offer him your phone number and/or your email address, can you expect his help in educating you on matters of fitness, diet, and exercise? Clients, at least some of them, can further their understanding of all matters relative to fitness via e-mail. Good trainers should appreciate your interest in what you're receiving from him.

How does he monitor his client's training progress? Does he review his findings with you in person or by way of an e-mail?

What are his fees for his instruction? How does he count for broken and missed appointments? What happens if he is late or forgets your appointment?

If you approach your prospective teacher with a check list or questionnaire, you may save yourself from future problems. All matters that come to your mind regarding your training should be answered in a friendly manner and concern for you as his client. After all, it's your money and your training should be worth what the fees are! Good luck and best wishes for your progress in all matters of fitness.

# Strength Training

Before you become confused, strength training is also referred to as "bodybuilding," "resistance training," or "weightlifting." You can do it at home, in a gym, with or without barbells and dumbbells, with or without machines or just with your own body weight. It's basically "muscle medicine" but not in liquid form or in pills or capsules. It's also different than most medicines in that there are so few negative side effects. Another axiom is that strength training is as close to obtaining the "fountain of youth" as one can find! Let's list some of the benefits of strength training:

1. It increases your resistance to many chronic diseases and even the effects of aging. The benefits you'll get will include heart health, lower blood pressure, and help in reducing your chance of getting cancer.
2. It aids to improve the quality of sleep so that your body rests more completely than if you didn't exercise.
3. It is an aid in relieving stress as you are doing something very constructive for yourself.
4. You improve your digestion and elimination processes. At the same time it offers a better control over excess weight gain.
5. It helps to increase your energy, endurance, strength, flexibility and power. When you become "addicted" to training, you'll automatically be concerned about your diet.
6. Weight control; muscle tissue burns more calories than fat as it has a higher rate of

metabolism generated within the muscle tissues.

7. There is an increased production of endorphins which help to reduce pain.
8. Increased strength, muscle tone and size, and help in increasing ligament, and tendon strength.
9. Increases bone density as the load upon the bones rises to form more fracture resistance from falling.
10. Increased production of some important hormones such as testosterone and growth hormone. The higher the intensity of the exercising the greater the increased amount of these two hormones and also other hormones.
11. There is increased cardiovascular and pulmonary circulation from strenuous training.
12. Body fat decreases while saving muscle tissue at the same time. When people diet without exercising, about 25% of the weight loss is muscle tissue, and that is not what we want!
13. Exercising increases the percentage of lean muscle tissues.
14. There is a decrease of serum cholesterol.
15. Besides increasing flexibility there is also an increased range of motion.
16. Training for strength reduces sarcopenia.
17. It helps you to feel young, vibrant, strong, trim, and healthy.
18. It can help in reducing heart rate as your fitness improves.
19. It helps to prevent injury. When the muscles are strengthened along with their attachments to their joints, if you endure an injury, it will help heal it faster and speed up the recovery time.

20. It you participate in other sports, strength training will help you to improve the activity at a higher level. A more fit body can boost the extra power and energy needed to excel in any endeavor.
21. Improves your appearance and satisfaction as a result of strength training.

As your body composition improves (less fat, more muscle = improved metabolism) your energy and focus on your body will increase. Consider a man weighing 185 lbs. before starting bodybuilding. With a BMI (body mass index) of 30, he is classified as being obese. He has 55.5 lbs of fat and a lean body weight of 129.5 lbs. (consisting of bones, organs, water, muscle, skin, etc.). If he starts an effective strength training program and replaces 5 lbs. of fat with 5 lbs. of muscle, his weight is still 185 lbs. But by losing 5 lbs. of fat his lean body weight increases to 134.5 lbs. The net result is an increase in strength, muscle tone, and metabolism improvement, giving him a fit appearance. It also increases his motivation to continue on with his training and his outlook for goal achievements in strength training.

# Interval Training

Interval training is a variation of same-tempo or lighter training. It blends continuous training with intervals of more intense, short periods and it probably developed in Sweden during the 1930s. Finland had a world class runner by the name of Paavo Nurmi, and it was he who far outclassed the Swedish running team. The Finns also had other members of their team that caused the Swedes to lose track meets when competing with the Finnish team. The Swede's had a men's national team coach, Gosta Holmer, who was a one-time bronze medalist in the Olympic decathlon. He decided to imitate the Finns and use some of the teaching methods in running that Paavo Nurmi and the other team members used. The main characteristic of the Finnish team was to train their runners in short practices but of very high intensity, once a week. The Swedes called the technique, fartlek, which means "speed play" in Swedish. Holmer varied the fartlek by sending his runners out into the hills and fields of Sweden rather than having them run around a track. The team members would sprint toward far off trees or rocks and then let them rest while running at a slower speed for a while. This developed into a high intensity short period with slower running of a longer duration. It amounted to a sprint, rest, sprint, rest, etc. The speed and endurance of the Swedish runners improved immeasurably and they became very competitive with other world running teams.

Interval training can be used in bodybuilding and most other types of exercising. It results in time-saving, high-intensity, short periods followed by lower intensity, longer periods to allow for rest. The trainee can vary each of the short and longer training periods, according to his ability and physical conditioning. The result is faster progress and physical improvement in your training regime over the slower same-tempo methods.

Some of the benefits of interval training are:

1. More calories are burned because you'll exercise more vigorously. The higher the intensity the more calories consumed.
2. Your exercise period will be of shorter duration and keep your progress at a higher and faster rate.
3. No special equipment is necessary. If you walk, workout at home, or in a gym, you can do interval training. All you have to do is modify your current routine.
4. Your cardio-vascular fitness will improve so you'll be able to exercise longer and/or at higher intensity.
5. As you exercise at a higher intensity, your body will become firmer, stronger, and your metabolic rate will improve. Along with watching your diet and what you eat, your pot belly will be gone sooner rather than later. In other words, all the benefits of exercise will be yours, in spades.

What are the potential risks?

Do not attempt interval training if you have physical limitations and if you do, get you doctor's recommendations as to the type, frequency, and any other factors that he may tell you to follow. You may also ask a personal trainer for advice.

Also do not jump into this type of high intensity training without a measure of caution. Start slowly and build up your training as your stamina improves. Challenge yourself to vary the pace. You may be surprised by the results.

Suggestions:

Depending on the type of exercising you do, warm up the muscles you plan to work on during your exercise period. If you run, warm up with a jog around the track, or maybe twice around the track. Then do a short run, at a faster pace than your jog spend, are then a rest period at a slower jog rate. Alternate this method as your body responds. Remember, if you do what you always did, you'll always get what you've always got. That's a great way to develop a plateau in your exercise regime, and what you really want is to progress beyond the plateau limit. Push yourself if you want results!

# Breathing While Exercising

If exercise is basically movement carried to a higher level of intensity, doesn't breathing change too? Yes, definitely, because you are placing an increased load on the body and when you do that, you'll have an increased heart rate, a higher demand for oxygen, and numerous other changes that occur. Some inexperienced trainees start an exercise by holding their breath, as if they were going to dive into water and swim beneath the surface. Maybe that's for fish to do but not for a human needing a flow of air!

Holding one's air is called a Valsalva maneuver and can result in a dangerous jump in blood pressure and sometimes even bursting some of the blood vessels in your eyes and brain. This can result in visual disturbances and headaches. If you are a heavy lifter of weights, sometimes a temporary hold of breathing is natural. It may result in only minor and transient increased blood pressure. But experienced weight lifters know that a Valsalva maneuver can be harmful if carried out for longer periods of time and so they may do it only for a short time.

As a general rule you should breathe out on the hardest part of the movement and in when the easiest stage of the movement occurs. To state the general rule, exhale while lifting and inhale when lowering the weight. On the other hand, two stalwarts on strength training, namely Dr. Stuart McGill and the late Dr. Mel

Siff, stated that "careful instruction as to the technique of a given exercise will automatically result in the body responding with the optimal muscle recruitment strategy throughout the duration of the movement."
My interpretation - follows the general rule, always exhale on exertion and inhale on the easier stage of the exercise. The important point is to allow a constant inflow and outflow of air as the intensity increases without holding your breathe for extended periods of time.

Another method of breathing that worked for me when I used to jog was to breathe in and out in cadence with the song by Disney, "It's A Small World"

it's a world of laughter, a world or tears
its a world of hopes, it's a world of fear
there's so much that we share
that its time we're aware
its a small world after all

CHORUS:
its a small world after all
its a small world after all
its a small world after all
its a small, small world

There is just one moon and one golden sun
And a smile means friendship to everyone.
Though the mountains divide
And the oceans are wide
It's a small small world

## The Interrelated Components
## Of Fitness

Let's assume you have been working out for a year or
more and your progress in fitness seems to have
stalled. Weight seems to be harder to lose, the waist
is bigger than it should be, and the initial change in
your body has slowed to a snail's pace. It's time to
recognize what fitness is all about, how to obtain it
and how to improve where you live, mainly in YOUR
body. Consider the following facts:

1. The amount of energy in 1 lb. of fat is 3500
   calories. If the machine you use (i.e., a
   treadmill) has a heart rate monitor and you use
   it for 1/2 hour, maybe you'll burn off 300
   calories. Maybe! If you have a snack of
   cookies or ice cream, cake, etc., you'll realize
   that 300 calories amounts to next to nothing.
   So exercise is not the best way to lose fat. A
   proper diet is and what you have to consume
   so eat good food and leave the pastry at the
   market. Cut your portions roughly 50% but eat
   smaller meals more frequently. Six smaller
   meals spaced thought the day will keep your
   energy up and your hunger pains down.
2. Think of exercising on a regular basis to
   maintain your musculature and the health of all
   your organs. Exercising is like playing a violin.
   When you're new to the instrument, you'll
   "fiddle" with it. Keep at it and eventually
   beautiful "music" will be your reward. Don't
   think of exercise as drudgery, but as an item
   like food, water, and sleep. Weave it into your
   daily life and you'll look forward to each
   workout.

3. Developing your muscles helps you to lose fat. If you exercise on a regular basis you will increase your metabolic rate. As you add muscle to your body, you'll burn more fat because muscle tissue requires a lot of energy just to be a major part of your body. Less muscle = lower metabolic rate = less energy = more stored fat = your life as a couch potato (let's hope not)!
4. Be sure your diet is relatively free of highly processed foods, coke, pop, candy, pastry and most fast foods. You don't need calories without nutrition.
5. Have a high fiber diet. The Mediterranean Diet is an example of a food source with adequate fiber. Also try to have some protein with each meal. Drink plenty of fluids, but mostly water.
6. Do weight bearing exercises. As we grow older, our bones become weaker and with less density. Weight lifting, strength training, and bodybuilding are all good examples of weight bearing exercising.
7. Some people think that by reducing carbohydrates one will burn more fat. The problem is that when carbs are reduced in amount consumed, the rate of fat metabolism slows down and this is not what you want. Also, fat then is burned into acidic fat know as ketone. Ketones, in high amounts, are dangerous and are so acidic they can kill cells. As a result, fat loss slows and muscle tissue loss increases. This is not what you want as one of the real purposes of exercise is the building up of the muscles in your body. The answer is to continue to eat carbs, the right kind and that includes more of the complex

carbohydrates (fruits and vegetables) and less of the sugar containing-nutritionally deficient, calorie loaded junk food.

8. Vary your training to confuse your muscles. This will also help you to progress up the slope of fitness and not stagnate into a plateau of, "I'm not getting anywhere in my training - why?" Increase the intensity of your workouts by doing more reps with lower weight and fewer reps with more weight. The number of reps should be between 5 and 15. Increase the rate of your movements and/or slow them down but always do enough sets of each exercise to warm the muscles involved, increase the resistance in following sets, and work to failure in your final set.

9. To control blood sugar and help prevent type 2 diabetes, include some protein, fat and carbohydrate into each meal, eat smaller amounts of food, but attempt to keep the blood insulin level on an even keel. Insulin helps to maintain a more constant glucose blood level. That means no high sugar containing snacks, especially in large amounts. Think of regular exercise as your best medicine for sugar control!

# Training for Beginners

In this article on training we are concerned with bodybuilding with weights, barbells, dumbbells, machines, benches, stability balls, and, sometimes, elastic bands.  There are many other forms of exercise and maybe weights may not be your forte over a period of time.  The advantage of weight training is that you can work the entire body, or parts of the body, and include the benefits of leaner muscles, strength increases, and improvement in your metabolism while reducing the chances of many debilitating diseases.  You can include exercises for balancing, core strengthening, flexibility, agility, and weight reduction.  As you advance in the training process, you will notice improvement in sleeping, energy, digestion, etc.  The list can go on and on!
 You will come to the realization that the human being is a muscle machine designed for movement.  One gets in trouble by thinking rest heals all.  Usually exercise, rest, proper diet, and moderation in all aspects are the keys to healthful fitness - first & forever.

A physical exam is a good practice for all ages, and especially for seniors.  You should know where your body needs special attention, its weaker areas, and limited movement locations.  If you have knee problems, arthritis, balance problems, as well as heart and lung limitations, your doctor can advise you as to what, where and when your body will need special considerations.

To save you time and money, have a certified personal trainer develop an exercise program according to your desires, capabilities, and general health. Many, if not most, clients of a gym are poor exercise trainees. Their form is incorrect, they train with distractions (conversations with others, cell phones, and wasting time resting between sets of exercises) to an extent that their progress is hampered and goals are not obtained. Once you have experience in training you can go on your own and whether you progress, or not, is up to you. Remember this statement as it pertains to most everything you do in life.................It's not the time you put into this program as much as it is what you do during the time spent! Review a previous article on "Movement vs. Exercise". To work the entire body usually means doing exercises that affect the larger muscle groups. They are as follows:

1. Legs (calves, quadriceps, hamstrings).
2. Back (upper and lower back - from the neck to the lumbar region).
3. Chest (pecs, over the head extensions on a bench, side raises with dumbbells, chest pressing with both dumbbells and barbells).
4. Arms, upper/lower including biceps, triceps, forearms, dips, curls, with dumbbells and barbells).
5. Abs and core exercises using benches, stability balls, crunches, etc.
6. Cardio training on treadmills, elliptical trainers, running, step machines, stationery bikes.

Usually a period of 30-60 minutes for a workout is recommended and, if possible, 4 times/week. If this requires more time than you want to devote to your exercise programs, do a workout 2 times per week. You can start out with 1 set of each exercise and learn the proper form for each movement. 8 to 15 reps are usually suggested and as you progress you can do multiple sets of each exercise. Also try to allow about 1 week of rest for each of the muscle groups. Cardio can be done at the beginning or ending of each exercise period or on separate days.

Do at least 10 minutes of cardio and use whatever machine you like best. The exercises listed for the various areas can be divided by the number of times you wish to work out during the week. If cardio on a machine is difficult for you, then consider walking. As you progress in your walking routine, time yourself and try to increase your speed. Maybe you may include a little jogging along with your walking. Good for you!

With regard to how to do each exercise, you now have the benefit of the Internet. Apple and android phones, tablets, and computers have a lot of information on each exercise you may expect to do. You can see videos, diagrams, and pictures of exercises, starts and finishes. Check out the apps available for your type of phone. A picture or two of each exercise is static, and does not detail the proper form from start to finish. You'll get a lot more out of watching a video of someone demonstrating how to do what you plan to do rather than looking at a front and side view of any exercise.

# Training for Beginners - Part 2

To do the various exercises, either have a personal trainer show you how and what to do to work your entire body or view the websites listed below. If you look at a book or magazine you will probably see a view of the beginning and another view of the end of the exercise. You need to know the rate or tempo of how fast or slow you do the movements and videos are preferred to fixed, stationary pictures.

By going online or using apps on a cell phone, you'll see how to do each exercise and often with an explanation of each movement. Below are 4 websites showing exercises for the major groups of muscles and you can also check out apps for your smart phone.

1. www.exercise4weightloss.com
2. www.fitnessblender.com
3. www.fitnessmagzine.com
4. www.sparkpeople.com. This website will show you exercises using a
   stability ball and they describe a 15 minute ball workout on a video.

Proper breathing during exercising is very important and you should practice on doing it correctly. Inspiratory ventilation occurs in two forms: normal resting state (quiet) breathing and heavy (deep, forced) breathing. The full breaths are those that will super-oxygenate your hardworking muscles and produce the most efficient workout. These breaths are called "belly" breaths. Many times during a workout, you may have a tendency to hold your breath. Doing so can raise your blood pressure and strain other organs, particularly the heart. Proper control of your breathing pattern keeps your blood pressure down. It also keeps you more relaxed and focused. As you contract (flex) your muscles, you should exhale and inhale upon relaxation of those same muscles.

# Strength Training For Seniors

Are you a youngster of 65 or more years? Do you spend half of your time in a doctor's office and the rest of your waking hours making doctor appointments, picking up medications at a pharmacy, and complaining of pains here, there and everywhere? Well my dear friend, you need help.

Let's start off with an appointment at your doctor's office and tell him (her) that you want a checkup to determine what kinds of exercise he recommends. What, if any, are your limitations that you should be aware of to tell your trainer? Get a form, signed by the doctor, that you can participate in strength training and have him list any items that need special attention (i.e., heart problems, recent surgeries, arthritis, etc.).

If you will go to a gym and get an experienced personal trainer, he'll get you started after obtaining your goals, time allowed for training, how often you can work with him during the week, and any other information he may require. If you have experience exercising, let him know and what you did and when you last worked out on a regular basis. This is choice No. 1!

If you do everything on your own, please look at some of the best places to offer help in your exercise plan. Each of these sources you can find on your computer. Also, you can see videos or pictures with explanations of what and how to do the various exercises.  The recommended sources are listed below.

1. 10 Best YouTube channels for free fitness videos: http://mashable.com/2013/01/21/youtube-fitness-videos/.
2. Physical Activity: Strength training for older adults: Exercises Step 1. DNPAO/CDC.
3. http://weighttraining.about.com/od/weighttrainingforgroups/a/seniorsbell0708.htm
4. http://nihseniorhealth.gov/exerciseandphysicalactivityexercisestotry/strengthexercises/01.html

.

# Strength Training For Seniors
# A Research Report

As we age there are changes in our brains and total nervous system. More specifically, one of the basic components of our nerves are neurons. As muscles atrophy with age, as in sarcopenia, neurons lose size, their myelination and their ability to regenerate. Throughout the body these changes can lead to incoordination, accidents, falls, and trauma.

In the August 2014, vol 28-Issue 8; The Journal of Strength & Conditioning Research had an article entitled Resistance Exercise May Improve Spatial Awareness and Visual Reaction in Older Adults. The authors were trying to determine if strength training had any effect on cognitive and physical impairments. Aerobic exercise has exhibited positive effects on both cognitive and physical impairment on older adults. Presently there are few pharmacological treatments available. Aerobic exercise has been of value in improving the cognition and reaction of older people, but to determine the results from resistance training was the purpose of this study.

Twenty five healthy adults 60 years or older were volunteers and were free of recent surgeries, heart disease, pulmonary problems, and metabolic symptoms. There were no musculoskeletal injuries so, essentially, they were in reasonably good health for their age group.  They were divided into two groups, a control group of 12 individuals and a training group of 13 people.

Thee training programs completed 2 days of training to become familiarized with the exercises they were taught.  They had 2 resistance training sessions for a period of 6 weeks with at least 48 hours of rest between all training sessions to allow for recovery. Full body workouts were performed during each session with 7 or 8 exercises performed each day.
 The workouts were for 3 sets of each exercise and the number of repetitions were 8 -15.  All sessions were monitored by a certified strength and conditioning specialist.  The program followed the recommended guidelines for older adults by the American College of Sports Medicine and the national Strength and Conditioning Association.

The exercises performed by the training group include:

1. Leg extensions
2. Leg curls
3. Seated rows
4. Lat pull-downs
5. Modified squats
6. Modified split squats
7. Modified stiff-legged dead lifts
8. Biceps curls
9. Chest presses
10. Shoulder presses
11. Triceps extensions

12. Abdominals
13. Calf raises

Results and Interpretations of the analyses revealed that resistance exercise training was "likely beneficial" for improving spatial awareness and visual and physical reaction times. The improvement of the training group over the control group for each of the senses is as follows:

1. Spatial awareness; +40%
2. Visual reaction times; +14.6%
3. Physical reaction times; +14%

According to the authors of this study, "The results of this study support the use of resistance exercise as a means to potentially preserve or improve spatial awareness and visual and physical reaction times in older adults. Both spatial awareness and reaction are essential to accident avoidance in everyday living because they enable the individual to perceive and react to the surrounding environment."

# Sarcopenia

Sarcopenia is characterized by a decrease of the size of the muscles which causes weakness and frailty. This loss may be caused by different cellular mechanisms than those that cause muscle atrophy. During sarcopenia, there is a replacement of muscle fibers with fat and an increase in fibrosis. An excellent article from WebMD follows this introduction.

"From the time you are born to around the time you turn 30, your muscles grow larger and stronger. But at some point in your 30s, you begin to lose muscle mass and function, a condition known as age-related sarcopenia or sarcopenia with aging. People who are physically inactive can lose as much as 3% to 5% of their muscle mass per decade after age 30. Even if you are active, you will still experience some muscle loss.

Although there is no generally accepted test or specific level of muscle mass for sarcopenia diagnosis, any loss of muscle mass is of consequence, because loss of muscle means loss of strength and mobility. Sarcopenia typically accelerates around age 75 -- although it may happen in people age 65 or 80 -- and is a factor in the occurrence of frailty and the likelihood of falls and fractures in older adults.

Although sarcopenia is mostly seen in people who stay physically inactive throughout life suggests there are other factors involved in the development of sarcopenia.

The primary treatment for sarcopenia is exercise. Specifically, resistance training or strength training -- exercise that increases muscle strength and endurance with weights or resistance bands -- has been shown to be useful for both the prevention and treatment of sarcopenia.

Resistance training has been reported to positively influence the neuromuscular system, hormone concentrations, and protein synthesis rate. Research has shown that a program of progressive resistance training exercises can increase protein synthesis rates in older adults in as little as two weeks.

For optimal benefits with minimal risk of injury, the proper number, intensity, and frequency of resistance exercise is important. For that reason, you should work with an experienced physical therapist or trainer to develop an exercise plan.

Although drug therapy is not the preferred treatment for sarcopenia, a few medications are under investigation. They include:

Urocortin II. This peptide has been shown to stimulate the release of a hormone called adrenocoticotropic hormone (ACTH) from the pituitary gland. Intravenous urocortin II has been shown to prevent muscle atrophy from being in a cast or taking certain medications; it has also been shown to cause muscle growth in healthy rats. But its use for building muscle mass in humans has not been studied and is not recommended.

Hormone Replacement Therapy (HRT). When a woman's production of hormones is diminished at menopause, hormone replacement therapy has been shown to increase lean body mass, reduce abdominal fat short-term, and prevent bone loss. However, in recent years there has been controversy surrounding the use of HRT due to increased risk of certain cancers and other serious health problems among HRT users.

Other treatments under investigation for sarcopenia include testosterone supplementation, growth hormone supplementation, and medication for treatment of metabolic syndrome (insulin-resistance, obesity, hypertension, etc.).  If found useful, all of these would complement the effects of resistance exercise, not replace them."

The material above is another good reason to include strength training as an important
part of your life.

# Muscular Fitness vs. Body Weight

**What's more important in
helping to prevent heart disease?
Answer; Muscular Fitness**

Exercise helps to prevent many chronic diseases that affect humans and heart disease is one of them. You have heard of cholesterol as being one of the factors and there are two types of cholesterol; HDL, the "good kind" and LDL, "the bad kind" of cholesterol. When there are high levels of HDL, it has been found to be effective in preventing heart disease. Exercise can increase HDL levels.

Researchers at UCLA have also found that the quality and function of the HDL are as important as its quantity. They tested 3 groups of young men as follows:

1. Overweight untrained with BMI's of 30 or higher. BMI is a test of body fat on an individual and 30 or above is considered obese.
2. Overweight but trained with BMI's of 29. They exercised 4 or more days per week doing strength training.
3. Lean trained with BMI's of 24. They also did strength training 4 or more times per week.

The results of their research are as follows:

1. The HDL function was significantly better in both of the trained groups compared with the overweight untrained group. They also found that the HDL function in the overweight trained group was not much different from that of the lean trained group.
2. The result of muscular fitness is more important than body weight for HDL functionality. Thus the functionality could be a mechanism by which resistance training (a.k.a. strength training) may decrease the risk of cardiovascular disease.
3. It was also noted that some hormonal and metabolic parameters were related to HDL functionality.
4. The high HDL function correlated with lower oxidized LDL, which is implicated in atherosclerosis, and also with higher testosterone levels. The latter may explained why low testosterone levels are associated with increased cardiovascular disease risk.

This study demonstrates that there is a relationship between HDL redox activity (an aspect of HDL function) and testosterone.

Reference; Roberts, C.K., et al, Untrained young men have dysfunctional HDL compared with strength-trained men irrespective of body weight status. J. Applied Physiology (1985), 2013, 4(4): p.1043-9

# The Couch Potato

The usual potato is planted into the ground, and given a delicious dose of fertilizer and water. They grow only in Idaho, and gradually turn into an oblong mass of carbohydrate. They ripen in the sun to turn a golden brown color.

A couch potato is a different species of potato, and they come from a fertilized egg found in the human female. As a youngster, they cry, make pee-pee, poop and cause many sleepless nights all around the globe, even in Seattle. After a while, they crawl, fall, and bawl. As they age, they eventually learn how to balance on two legs, like little gorillas. When they patrol their home they come upon a bed-like object called a couch. The couch in most homes is within easy viewing distance of the television set. Using their youth, strength, and growing legs, they perch themselves on the couch where they spend almost all of their life.

The diet of the couch potato resembles that of their cousins as it is an offshoot of fertilizer called, trash. It consists of sugar, sugar products, high fructose corn syrup, pastry, cake, cookies, etc., etc. With the TV turned on they lay flat on the couch and stuff themselves with trash. What little muscle they had before "couching", it atrophies, and their little hands can no longer hold their cell phones. Soon, with little movement and a lot of trash, they "round out" and roll off the couch. Eventually, they are involved with some chronic potato disease and succumb to it.

The moral of the story is that you do not want to live like a couch potato, so get off your butt and move around. Try good food and you'll live a happy, healthy life so you can get to the gym more often!

# Your Diet - The Simple Approach

Let's assume you don't want to count calories or follow any strict diet plan.  You may be eating in a restaurant or be invited to a friend's home.  Let's also follow the magic KISS formula (Keep It Simple, Stupid).  Follow a few simple rules even dummies can remember!

1.      If it doesn't come from the earth or have a mother, don't eat it.  Note: If you're a vegetarian, this may not be for you.

2.      If it's stuffed with, or has a lot of sugar in it, pass it by.  Note:  Sugar includes table sugar, maltose, dextrose, high fructose corn syrup, or fructose. Sugar is an irritant to your body and has no nutritional value.

3.      If it's highly processed, highly salted or has a lot of spice added, pass it by. This is true of most packaged soups, and processed meat items such as baloney, bacon, and similar items at your favorite market.

4.      Eat at least 25 grams of fiber for women and 38 grams for men each day. Along with fiber consume about 8 glasses of liquids each day.  Please, pass on soft drinks, beer, and alcohol as they all have extra calories with little or no nutritional value.  Fiber and liquids work together to aid regular bowel movements, without straining!

5. Try to add fruits and vegetables either with meals or as snacks.

6. Avoid stuffing at meal time by keeping your portions smaller than usual and by adding simple snacks half way between your breakfast, lunch and dinner.

7. Eat protein foods with each meal as they tend to rebuild your body and reduce hunger feelings.

8. Check food labels and stay away from foods with a lot of calories, trans-fats and saturated fats.

9. Don't be misled by energy drinks. The only way you can get energy is by eating a good, nutritional diet. Energy drinks are really mislabeled. They are stimulants!

If you can follow all of the above, have a PO Day twice each month. PO = pig out!

Whoopee, eat as you please but don't overdo your PO days.

# Diet & Facts You Should Know

In this book the Mediterranean Diet is highly recommended. It has an excellent history of providing good nutrition and helps to reduce the presence of many chronic diseases. It replaces junk foods with healthy carbohydrates, fats, and proteins. You will hear about all kinds of weight-loosing plans that stress either high or low fats, cutting out carbs, and little about proteins. Let's review some facts about the three macronutrients that should form the bulk of what you eat.

Proteins break down to form amino acids and there are 20 different amino acids. Of those 20, there are 9 essential amino acids and essential because they cannot be manufactured by your body. Therefore they must come from food sources such as meat, poultry, fish and dairy products. Eggs, milk, cottage cheese, and yogurt are examples of dairy foods. Protein can be found in vegetables like soybeans, sun-dried
tomatoes, winged beans, and baby lima beans.

Proteins are the building blocks of our organs, muscles, cells and most of our body fluids. Their main function is to build and repair body tissues and structures. Protein is involved in the synthesis of hormones, enzymes, and other regulatory peptides.

Fats (or lipids) are the most concentrated source of energy in our diet. A gram of fat yields approximately 9 calories when oxidized, furnishing more than twice the calories per gram of carbohydrates or proteins. Each gram of protein and carbohydrate delivers 4 calories per gram. Besides providing energy, the fats act as carriers for the fat-soluble vitamins A, D, E, and K. Fats also act as precursors to hormones, cellular membrane structure and function, regulation and excretion of nutrients in the cells, insulating the body from environmental temperature changes and in preserving body heat. They also act in prolonging the digestive process by slowing the stomach's secretions of hydrochloric acid, creating a longer-lasting sensation of fullness after a meal.

Carbohydrates are compounds containing carbon, hydrogen and oxygen. They are classified as sugars (simple), starches (complex) and fiber. Simple sugars are also referred to as monosaccharides and examples include glucose (blood sugar), fructose (fruit sugar) and galactos. Disaccharides are two sugar units and include sucrose (common sugar), lactose (milk sugar) and maltose.

Carbohydrates (sometimes referred to as "carbs") are the chief source of energy for all body functions and muscular exertion. They help to regulate the digestion and utilization of protein and fat.

Complex carbs, such as fiber, provide bulk in the diet, thus increasing the satiety value of foods. They come in two forms; soluble and insoluble fiber. Soluble fiber absorbs water and forms a thick gel-like consistency that expands to traps certain nutrients and slows the digestive process. Because of this, sugar is absorbed into the bloodstream more slowly, causing fewer spikes in blood sugar and thus helps in preventing diabetes. This soluble fiber also prevents some of the cholesterol in the food from being absorbed and it also inhibits cholesterol production in the liver.

Insoluble fiber does not absorb water and provides the bulk that speeds the digestive process and thus helps to prevent constipation. This type of fiber also helps to remove heavy metals and other toxins from the large intestine. The peels of fruits and vegetables and the bran, or outer covering of seeds are examples of insoluble fibers. Good sources are fruits, whole grains, vegetables and brown rice.

From the information given here, you can see that each of these three macronutrients have definitive functions, specific to the protein, fat and carbohydrate groupings. The Mediterranean Diet is structured to provide a balance, in proportion, to the three nutrient groups in a structured and proven manner.

# Nutrition - A Recommended Diet

Of our four pillars of health and fitness, namely Exercise, Rest, Sleep, and now, Nutrition (Diet), let's see what makes sense. Pick up almost any magazine or newspaper and you'll see many, many, diet recommendations. Why do so many people look to diet as a means of losing weight? Well, exercise alone is a poor method of losing our "pot" bellies. If one eats the wrong foods, or too much of most any food (s), you'll pack on the pounds. If you only diet without exercising, you can lose weight but you'll also loose muscle. That's a no-no for a fitness buff.

What really matters is not so much what one weighs but what the composition of the person's body is. There are percentages of fat, muscle, etc. that are recommended. Much more information can be found at Monica Mullica's address: http://www.mowifit.com/Its_your_body_composition_not_bodyweight_that_matters.pdf. Monica is a nationally recognized expert on nutrition and exemplifies her appearance on the bodybuilder physique that she so successfully displays. The article she wrote is quite lengthy so you might want to go to the Summery at the end of her composition.

So let's see what makes for a healthy diet. For any diet to be successfully followed, it should not be too rigid or complicated in its structure. It should allow for good nutritional value, few if any saturated fats, no trans fats, sweets (pastry, bagels, surgery products), with much more fresh fruit and vegetables than most dieters eat.  A quick rule of thumb is "If it has a mother or if it comes from the earth, it's OK to eat."  Read the labels as they are of considerable help in determining the food's nutritional content.

After considering the present knowledge of healthful diets, I would recommend the Mediterranean Diet and to get a good perspective of how it works, look at one of its locations, the Mayo Clinic. The Mayo Clinic displays a pyramid of the diet. The address at the Mayo Clinic Mediterranean Diet is: http://www.mayoclinic.org/Mediterranean-diet/art-20047801

# The Mediterranean Diet

One of the best characteristics of the Mediterranean Diet is that it is easy to follow, and allows enough variance in food choices to keep you interested in its basic design.
It includes more fruit and vegetables, fewer fats, especially the saturated variety, more olive oil, nuts and beans, healthy whole grains, and smaller amounts of dairy and meat.
They even allow some red wine.

How does it work?

The diet is designed to reduce the chance of getting heart disease by lowering blood pressure and cholesterol. It may also help to in avoiding some cancers and chronic diseases.

For weight loss they recommend a reduction of processed products such as pastry, donuts, high fructose corn syrup, sugary items, and most 'junk foods' Also try to stay away from fried foods and most anything else that has calories but little or no nutrition.

Recommended foods include low-fat yogurt, poultry, cheese, and eggs. Try to eat fish, of the more oily variety, like salmon, at least twice a week. Make your salads with sunflower seeds, avocados, virgin olive oil, most nuts, and a touch of herbs and spices to add flavor. Fresh foods should replace packaged foods or packaged meals.

A well rounded diet, consumed in moderate proportions, affords a good supply of protein, carbohydrates, and fat. You'll get all the vitamins and minerals you'll require from this meal plan. As an added measure, a multi-vitamin-mineral tablet once a day can be your form of insurance!

A sensible diet such as the Mediterranean Diet, along with regular exercise, rest and sleep, should afford a good opportunity to lower your odds of getting diabetes, osteoporosis, depression and Alzheimer's. Even you waist line will thank you.

What really matters is not so much what one weighs but what the composition of the person's body is. There are percentages of fat, muscle, etc. that are recommended. Much more information can be found at Monica Mollica's address: http://www.mowifit.com/Its_your_body_composition_not_bodyweight_that_matters.pdf. Monica is a nationally recognized expert on nutrition and exemplifies her appearance on the bodybuilder physique that she so successfully displays. The article she wrote is quite lengthy so you might want to go to the Summery at the end of her composition.

So let's see what makes for a healthy diet. For any diet to be successfully followed, it should not be too rigid or complicated in its structure. It should allow for good nutritional value, few if any saturated fats, no trans fats, sweets (pastry, bagels, surgery products), with much more fresh fruit and vegetables than most dieters eat. A quick rule of thumb is "If it has a mother or if it comes from the earth, it's OK to eat." Read the labels as they are of considerable help in determining the food's nutritional content.

After considering the present knowledge of healthful diets, I would recommend the Mediterranean Diet and to get a good perspective of how it works, look at one of its locations, the Mayo Clinic. The address at the Mayo Clinic Mediterranean Diet is: http://www.mayoclinic.org/Mediterranean-diet/art-20047

# The Mediterranean Diet

The Mediterranean Diet suggests the following:

1.  Eating primarily plant-based foods, such as fruits and vegetables, whole grains,

    Legumes and nuts
2.  Replacing butter with healthy fats, such as olive oil
3.  Using herbs and spices instead of salt to flavor food
4.  Limiting red meat to no more than a few times a month
5.  Eating fish and poultry at least twice a week
6.  Drinking red wine in moderation (optional)

The diet also recognizes the importance of being physically active and enjoying meals with family and friends.

Focus on fruits, vegetables, nuts and grains

The Mediterranean diet traditionally includes fruits, vegetables and grains. For example, residents of Greece average six or more servings a day of antioxidant-rich fruits and vegetables.

Grains in the Mediterranean region are typically whole grain and usually contain very few unhealthy trans-fats, and bread is an important part of the diet. However, throughout the Mediterranean region, bread is eaten plain or dipped in olive oil — not eaten with butter or margarine, which contains saturated or trans fats.

Nuts are another part of a healthy Mediterranean diet. Nuts are high in fat, but most of the fat is healthy. Because nuts are high in calories, they should not be eaten in large amounts — generally no more than a handful a day. For the best nutrition, avoid candied or honey-roasted and heavily salted nuts

Choose healthier fats

The focus of the Mediterranean diet isn't on limiting total fat consumption, but rather on choosing healthier types of fat. The Mediterranean diet discourages saturated fats and hydrogenated oils (trans-fats), both of which contribute to heart disease.

The Mediterranean diet features olive oil as the primary source of fat. Olive oil is mainly monounsaturated fat — a type of fat that can help reduce low-density lipoprotein (LDL) cholesterol levels when used in place of saturated or trans fats. "Extra-virgin" and "virgin" olive oils (the least processed forms) also contain the highest levels of protective plant compounds that provide antioxidant effects.

Canola oil and some nuts contain the beneficial linolenic acid (a type of omega-3 fatty acid) in addition to healthy unsaturated fat. Omega-3 fatty acids lower triglyceride, decrease blood clotting, and are associated with decreased incidence of sudden heart attacks, improve the health of your blood vessels, and help moderate blood pressure. Fatty fish — such as mackerel, lake trout, herring, sardines, albacore tuna and salmon — are rich sources of omega-3 fatty acids. Fish is eaten on a regular basis in the Mediterranean diet.

What about wine?

The health effects of alcohol have been debated for many years, and some doctors are reluctant to encourage alcohol consumption because of the health consequences of excessive drinking. However, alcohol — in moderation — has been associated with a reduced risk of heart disease in some research studies.

The Mediterranean diet typically includes a moderate amount of wine, usually red wine. This means no more than 5 ounces (148 milliliters) of wine daily for women of all ages and men older than age 65 and no more than 10 ounces (296 milliliters) of wine daily for younger men. More than this may increase the risk of health problems, including increased risk of certain types of cancer.

If you're unable to limit your alcohol intake to the amounts defined above, if you have a personal or family history of alcohol abuse, or if you have heart or liver disease refrain from drinking wine or any other alcohol.

Putting it all together

The Mediterranean diet is a delicious and healthy way to eat. Many people who switch to this style of eating say they'll never eat any other way. Here are some specific steps to get you started:

Eat your veggies and fruits — and switch to whole grains. A variety of plant foods should make up the majority of your meals. They should be minimally processed — fresh and whole are best. Include veggies and fruits in every meal and eat them for snacks as well. Switch to whole-grain bread and cereal, and begin to eat more whole-grain rice and pasta products. Keep baby carrots, apples and bananas on hand for quick, satisfying snacks. Fruit salads are a wonderful way to eat a variety of healthy fruit.

Go nuts. Nuts and seeds are good sources of fiber, protein and healthy fats. Keep almonds, cashews, pistachios and walnuts on hand for a quick snack. Choose natural peanut butter, rather than the kind with hydrogenated fat added. Try blended sesame seeds (tahini) as a dip or spread for bread.

Pass on the butter. Try olive or canola oil as a healthy replacement for butter or margarine. Lightly drizzle it over vegetables. After cooking pasta, add a touch of olive oil, some garlic and green onions for flavoring. Dip bread in flavored olive oil or lightly spread it on whole-grain bread for a tasty alternative to butter. Try tahini as a dip or spread for bread too.

Spice it up. Herbs and spices make food tasty and can stand in for salt and fat in recipes.

Go fish. Eat fish at least twice a week. Fresh or water-packed tuna, salmon, trout, mackerel and herring are healthy choices. Grill, bake or broil fish for great taste and easy cleanup. Avoid breaded and fried fish.

Rein in the red meat. Limit red meat to no more than a few times a month. Substitute fish and poultry for red meat. When choosing red meat, make sure it's lean and keep portions small (about the size of a deck of cards). Also avoid sausage, bacon and other high-fat, processed meats.

Choose low-fat dairy. Limit higher fat dairy products, such as whole or 2 percent milk, cheese and ice cream. Switch to skim milk, fat-free yogurt and low-fat cheese.

# The Mediterranean Diet
## A Summary of Research Studies

1. A study from researchers from the Harvard School of Public Health (HSPH) and Cambridge Health Alliance (CHA) and was published online in PLOS ONE on February 4, 2014. The study shows that promoting Mediterranean-style diets could have significant health benefits for young, working populations. The diet was rich in fish, nuts, vegetables, and fruits.

2. A study was published in Circulation, 2014 September 29, pii (Epub ahead of print) (Lahey R et al.) This involved an animal study at the University of Illinois where two diets were compared, The diet fat found in animal fats, dairy and palm oil was the first diet that was delivered to beating rat hearts with heart failure. The second diet was dietary fat found in olive oil. The first diet fed to the rats caused continued failing, with depressed fat metabolism and storage. The second diet treated hearts greatly improved, with restored fat content in cells, improved contraction, and normalized fat metabolism genes. The scientists observed the hearts treated with the olive oil noticed the fat content, turnover, and oxidation the failing hearts "were

indistinguishable from those of the healthy heart."

3. A study was published in Progress in Cardiovascular Diseases, 2014 September 4. Pii S00-0620 (14) 00133-9 (Epub ahead of print). Mediterranean diet decreases risk of mouth cancer. The studies involved 768 people with incident cases of mouth cancer, and 2078 people with no history of mouth cancer. The scientists found that diets high in fruits and vegetables have shown strong evidence that those with the highest adherence to the Mediterranean Diet had the lowest risk for mouth cancer.

A number of other studies found that the Mediterranean Diet:
   1. Decreases diabetes risk
   2. May decrease asthma in children
   3. There is a long tern improvement in vascular function after the Mediterranean diet.
   4. Can protect against breast cancer
   5. Decreases risk of frailty in ageing adults
   6. Reduces risk of cognitive decline
   7. Vegetarian diets have lower greenhouse gas emissions and lower mortality rates

# Sugar & Spice

# Makes Nothing Nice

My dad was a dentist and I followed him into dentistry a number of years after he began his practice. We both had the knowledge that sugar was bad for teeth as it is a major contributor to dental caries (tooth decay). Subsequently, medical research has found that sugar is bad news for one's health. Much has been written about the adverse effects of excessive sugar in the diet. Fortunately, the addition of fluoride to drinking water has reduced caries substantially and most of our palatable water is fluoridated nationwide. Although we have sugar substitutes there are so many forms of sugar that it is a common additive in too many dishes and drinks. Consider that we have table sugar, cane sugar, glucose, maltose, fructose, lactose, high fructose corn syrup, etc., etc.

Worldwide we consume about 500 extra calories a day from sugar. If you follow a diet that includes 500 extra calories a day then this amounts to gaining a pound a week. Let's look at how sugar affects your health:

> 1.    A high sugar diet makes us fat if you don't burn it off. Exercise is great for the body but it's easier to drop fat by dieting. The amount of calories that you get from exercising

on a treadmill may amount to 300 calories but if you eat a few cookies or some cake, going through 300 calories can be consumed in minutes!

2.      Sugar can accelerate the aging process. There is a relationship between glucose consumption and the aging of our cells.  Sugar can affect the aging of your brain as found in a 2009 study.

3.      There is evidence that excess sugar consumption is linked to deficiencies in memory and overall cognitive health in a study done in 2012.  Tests on rats showed similar findings as shown in a study done in 2009.

4.      Sugar hides in many of the foods we eat daily.  These include fat-free dressings, beverages, tomato sauce, tonic water, marinates, crackers, cake and even bread.

5.      Sugar and alcohol have similar toxic liver effects on the body .An article in *Nature* magazine came up with the idea that limitations and warnings should be placed on sugar similar to warnings that we see on alcohol.  There is evidence that fructose and glucose can cause liver damage.

6.      Excess sugar may shorten your life.  In a study done in 2013, an estimated 180,000 deaths worldwide may be attributed to sweetened beverage consumption.  Just in the United States the count is 25,000 deaths in 2010.  The researcher's state that deaths occurred due to the association with sugar-sweetened beverages and chronic disease risk as found in diabetes, heart disease and cancer.

7.     Sugar "addiction" may be genetic.  A study of 579 individuals showed that those who had genetic changes in the hormone called ghrelin consumed more sugar (and alcohol) than those that had no gene variation.  Ghrelin signals the brain that you're hungry.  It seems to be that the genetic components that affect the release of ghrelin may have a lot to do with whether or not you seek to enhance a neurological reward system through your addiction to sugar.

8.     Sugar can be harmful to cardiac health.  The American Heart Association states that there is strong evidence that sugar can affect the pumping mechanism of your heart and could increase the risk of heart failure.  The study pinpointed a molecule from sugar (G6P) was responsible for the changes in the muscle protein of the heart.

9.     Sugar may be involved in cancer production and could affect cancer survival.  In the metabolism of carbohydrates, which includes sugar, insulin helps to control the amount of sugar in the blood.  If one eats a lot of sugar, the insulin can become resistant over time and not function to monitor a healthy level of blood glucose.  There are studies that found negative associations between high sugar intake and survival rates in both breast cancer patients and colon cancer patients.

10.    It's important to note that simple sugars coming from fruit are less concerning given their high amounts of disease-fighting compounds and fiber.

# What Happens During Sleep?

As the afternoon wears on, we realize that in a few more hours it will be sleep time. After all, we either get up early to take the kids to school, go to work, shop for food, clothes or whatever and however we spend the day. It all requires energy and, like your cell phone, it needs charging at night. So sleep time is when your body rests and restores its energy levels. It is a state that affects both your physical and mental well-being. If you've had a good night's sleep, you'll feel ready to do the things that fill your day with activity and have enough energy left over to spend with your family or talk to friends. Let's look at what sleep involves and learn a little bit about its four stages.

Stage 1. Sleep studies show a reduction in activity between wakefulness and stage 1 sleep. The eyes are closed but the depth of sleep is such that if one is awakened, it is early sleep and the person may feel as if he or she has not slept. This period may last for 5 - 10 minutes.

Stage 2. Studies at this time now show intermittent peaks and valleys, and the waves and either positive or negative. There are spontaneous periods of increased muscle tone mixed with periods of muscle relaxation. Also, the heart rate slows and the body temperature decreases. When this happens, the body prepares to enter deep sleep.

Stage 3 and 4. The brain waves are known as slow or delta wave sleep. If awakened in these stages one may feel disoriented for a few minutes. Most of the beneficial effects of sleep can be found in stage three and four. As sleep deepens and becomes more intense, it progresses to stage 4. After about 90 minutes from entering the sleeping stages, REM sleep follows for about 10 minutes. Each REM recurring deepens and lengthens so that as it progresses, sleep is more intense.

Stage 3 is characterized by the release of the human growth hormone, or HGH. Blood rushes from the brain to the muscles to initiate recovery and to re-energize your body. Up to 70% or the production of HGH may occur in stage three and this is also when the immune function and normal glucose metabolism is supported.

Stage 4 is also known as "rapid-eye-movement sleep" or REM. This is when we dream, our arms and legs are still, and the total body seems paralyzed. It is also when the sleep is associated with learning and memory retention. The body repairs and regenerates tissues, builds muscle and bone, and strengthens the immune system. The day's information is kind of like a computer uploading information and clearing its RAM onto the hard drive.

Some of the important benefits of slow-wave sleep are:

HGH is produced and if you want to get stronger and faster, then you need your body to maximize the natural production of HGH. If sleep is not adequate in time or depth or if exercise is not intense enough to make changes, there will be little HGH produced.

There is a suppression of cortisol. Cortisol helps the body cope with the stress of daily life. When there are high levels of cortisol in the night it helps to create insulin resistance and this is linked to disorders such as Type 2 diabetes, as well as memory loss and cognitive impairment. This process will throw off your body's ability to process glucose throughout the day.

There is a suppression of the sympathetic nervous system in favor of the parasympathetic nervous system. The sympathetic nervous system is what is activated under stress, whereas the parasympathetic nervous system is what the body activates to recover and recuperate.

During deep sleep there is a release of prolactin; which is necessary for proper immune system function.

A good night's sleep is often the best way to help you cope with stress, solve problems or recover from illness.

Summarized; insufficient REM sleep has a negative impact on the brain as a whole and causes it to function abnormally. Therefore, get your sleep!

# The What and Why of a "Sleep Study"

After a workout your muscles may be a little sore, depending on the intensity of your exercising. High intensity training (HIT) causes some damage to the muscle fibers. There may be some fibers that are torn, some microscopic bleeding, and maybe soreness of the muscles. Sounds bad, huh? Not really. When you sleep your muscles heal, regenerate, and are strengthened. In other words, they are slightly firmer and healthier than before the workout. And the better and deeper your sleep is, the faster you progress in your fitness goals.

There are a number of problems serious enough to reduce the time and depth of your sleep. Just as you improve your form and intensity of your exercises, you should try to improve your sleeping period. Sleep studies are tests that record what happens to your body during sleep. They are performed in specialized rooms equipped with medical devices that record multiple body functions during sleep. Thus, brain activity, eye movement, oxygen and carbon dioxide blood levels, heart rate and rhythm, breathing rate and rhythm, the flow of air through your nose and mouth, snoring, body muscle movements and chest and belly movements are all recorded. This is an over-night visit to some sleep lab such as in the hospital or sleep lab privately owned by a doctor or group of doctors. Polysomnography is this type of sleep study and is usually recommended in cases of sleep apnea, seizure disorders, periodic limb movement disorders, insomnia, and narcolepsy.

Some of the sleep studies can help diagnose or rule out a number of disorders and they include:

1. Sleep apnea
2. Periodic limb movement disorders related to sleep, including twitching of the feet, arms, or legs during sleep
3. Seizure disorders
4. Insomnia caused by depression, hunger, physical discomfort, stress or some other problem
5. Extreme daytime tiredness, such as narcolepsy
6. Bruxism or grinding of the teeth during sleep
7. Shift work sleep disorder because of working period changes
8. Stages of sleep, non-rapid eye movement (NREM) and rapid eye movement sleep (REM)
9. Sleepwalking, night, terrors, or bed-wetting, each one a nighttime behavior problem

So after reading some or all of the above, how about some shut-eye?

# Sleep Apnea

One of the abnormalities of healthy sleeping is sleep apnea. This occurs when the upper airway is intermittently narrowed during sleep, causing breathing to be difficult or completely blocked. These can be brief interruptions in breathing during sleep, or they are of varying length, throughout the sleeping period. It can also be called obstructive sleep apnea, the most common form, and if it continues on without treatment, it can raise the risk for stroke, cardiovascular disease and heart attacks.

A recent study supported by the National Heart, Lung, and Blood Institute (NHLBI) of the National Institutes of Health (NIH) recently published a report in the open-access Journal of PLoS Medicine. The study consisted of more than 6,000 men and women aged 40 years and older who had no sleep apnea or had mild, moderate, or severe sleep apnea. After an average of eight years, the participants who had severe sleep apnea at enrollment were one and one-half times more likely to die from any cause, regardless of age, gender, race, or weight, or whether they were current or former smokers or had other medical ailments such as high blood pressure, heart disease, or diabetes. Other findings linked untreated sleep apnea with overweight and obesity, and diabetes. Untreated sleep apnea contributes to excessive daytime sleepiness, which lowers the performance in the workplace and at school, and increases the risk of injuries and death from drowsy driving and other accidents.

It has been estimated that more than 12 million adult Americans are believed to have sleep apnea, and most are not diagnosed or treated. Treatment is aimed at restoring normal breathing and includes lifestyle changes, surgery, mouthpieces, and breathing devices, such as continuous positive airway pressure, or CPAP. Treatment routines can help to restore sleep-related quality of life and performance.

Another study published in the endocrine Society's Journal of Clinical Endocrinology & Metabolism (JCEM) states that obstructive sleep apnea may raise the risk of osteoporosis, particularly among women or older individuals. One of the study's anchors, Kai-Jen Tien, MD, of Chi Mei Medical Center in Tainan, Taiwan states, "when sleep apnea periodically deprives the body of oxygen, it can weaken bones and raise the risk of osteoporosis. The progressive condition can lead to bone fractures, increased medical costs, reduced quality of life and even death." "As more and more people are diagnosed with obstructive sleep apnea worldwide, both patients and health care providers need to be aware of the heightened risk of developing other conditions," Tien said, "We need to pay more attention to the relationship between sleep apnea and bone health so we can identify strategies to prevent osteoporosis."

# Sleeping Positions Can Affect Sleep

Comes bedtime, you're tired and you want a good night's sleep. Tomorrow is a busy day and you also have a social engagement at 7:00 P.M. If you are an active sleeper, meaning you probably toss and turn during the night, it's not easy to answer, "What's the best sleeping position"?

A study was done as to how American's sleep. Here's the breakdown; 63% sleep on their side, 14% on their back, 16% on their stomach and most combine combinations of at least 2 or 3 positions during the night. What really counts is how much energy you have in the late afternoon and if you usually get between 6 and 8 hours of sleep time.

There are situations of pain in the neck, back or side that help to determine in what position you should start your evening's slumber. Some people have an acid reflux problem and they usually do better elevating their head or raise the end of the bed where the head is positioned. You can do that with special blocks of wood that are elevated so you put one block on the right and the other block on the left side of the bed.

For neck pain, don't sleep on your stomach or use a thick pillow because you can cause tension in the neck muscles. Try to keep your neck in a neutral position, following the line of your back laying flat on the bed.

If your shoulders are causing pain, don't sleep on the side that causes you pain.  A good trick is to use a large pillow next to you and place your arm over it. It's like sleeping with another person and you are hugging them.  This elevates and supports the sore arm helping to relieve your pain.

If your back aches, depending where the pain is, you might feel better with a rolled-up
towel under your knees to give them support.  On your side you can use a pillow under your top-most leg if it relieves your pain.

If your feet bother you, as in plantar fasciitis, try to find a relaxing position for your ankles and feet.  Plantar fasciitis is an inflamed sore area on the bottom of the foot.  It can arise by running or have poor arch support.  Also try not to tuck in the foot end of the sheet too tightly.   Pressure on the toes may be due to too little room at the foot-end of the bed when sheets are not loose enough for foot comfort.

# Exercise;
# How it affects your hormones

Hormones are produced by specific organs of the body and they travel to their receptor sites through the blood stream. Once received, they perform and are involved in many physiological and chemical activities. They help regulate metabolism, digestion, sleep, respiration, excretion, stress, growth and are involved in all functions of living. What's really important is that each hormone is very specific in what it does.

When a hormone has bonded to a receptor cell, it can send messages to the cell and tell it, and effectively the entire body, to perform a specific function. A few of the hormones are listed here as well as how they function.

Epinephrine and norepinephrine, produced in the adrenal cortex, are responsible for regulation of the cardiac output. When you exercise there is a release of both of these hormones as a result of the stress placed on the body. There is also the increase in the blood pressure that is experienced during exercise; along with the constricting effect that epinephrine has on the blood vessels. There is an increase in blood pressure due to the tension of the blood vessels as a result of the norepinephrine.

The amount of these hormones secreted is dependent upon the level of activity. As the intensity of the exercise increases there is more hormone secretion along with demands of more oxygen to afford the changes in bodily adaptation.

Both epinephrine and norepinephrine are responsible for the breaking down glycogen from the liver into glucose in the bloodstream. The demand for glucose is increased according to the intensity of physical activity

.

Vasopressin is released in order to reduce urinary excretion of water. This is to counteract the excretion of water by sweat when perspiration occurs. This is also to prevent dehydration caused by water loss. Vasopressin is also involved in keeping the blood plasma level within a varying range caused the exercising. This hormone helps to maintain a proper electrolyte balance so you don't cramp or experience other symptoms that can arise when you lose too many electrolytes.

Cortisol, also called hydrocortisone, is produced in the adrenal cortex, which is the outer part of each adrenal gland. After a stressful situation passes, cortisol tells the body what fat, protein or carbohydrates to burn and when to burn them and it depends on what kind of challenge you face. It can also take your fat, in the form of triglycerides, and move it to your muscle, or break down muscle and convert it into glycogen for more energy. An excess of cortisol can deconstruct bone and skin, leading to osteoporosis and easy bruising.

Cortisol can increase your cravings for high-fat, high-carb foods. It can also lower leptin levels and increase the levels of neuropeptide Y (NPY), a shift proven to stimulate appetite.

Testosterone comes from the testes, ovaries, and adrenal glands. In the male it is best known for the male sexual characteristics. The male androgens include testosterone, androstenedione, and dehydroepian- drosterone (DHEA). They are steroid hormones because their chemical structure is derived from cholesterol. They are known as anabolic steroids because there is a metabolic process that promotes tissue growth. They are active in stimulating the growth of muscle tissue. Exercise increases the testosterone availability as it does with human growth hormone (HGH).

Growth hormone is a chain of 191 amino acids. They can instruct the body to perform protein synthesis and cell transport. More of it is secreted in response to exercise.

Although many hormones are affected by exercise, testosterone, cortisol, and growth hormones are usually the big three that people are interested in.

# Hormones and Weight Control

Hormones are biochemical products produced by glands and there are approximately 50 of them in the human body but there will probably be more found as research progresses. They are transported by the circulatory system to distant target organs where they regulate many physiological and chemical activities. They help maintain metabolism, digestion, sleep, respiration, excretion, stress, growth and are involved in all functions of living.

With regard to weight control, Leptin, a hormone, is involved in body fat in that it is a strong suppressor of one's appetite. It is produced in fat cells. Leptin works with other hormones such as thyroid, cortisol, and insulin in determining how hungry you get, how fast it will burn off the food you eat, and if it will hang on to, or let go of weight. Leptin also helps to tap into fat stores and thereby reduce them. On the other hand, when leptin doesn't do its function properly, you keep eating because you never feel like you've had enough food. Leptin and insulin resistance go hand in hand. If you lose weight, your body will become more sensitive to leptin and it will start acting the way it was intended. Insulin is also more sensitive in normal weighted individuals. Obesity reduces sensitivity and is one of the causes of type 2 diabetes. In other words, leptin will help you to push away from the table and say, "I've had enough!" So control what you eat and the amount consumed to ward off obesity and diabetes.

Ghrelin, another hormone, tells your brain, "I'm hungry, let's eat!"  This hormone is produced in the stomach and upper intestine.  When you think about food, your gut releases ghrelin.  The positive side of ghrelin is the help it gives to the pituitary gland to release growth hormone.

The body chemistry is very complex but to keep it healthy you have choices in the food you eat, and the amount you gobble down once it gets past your teeth.  To keep your body healthy and trim, you have to have a basic sense of your diet, exercise, sleep, water and calorie consumption, stress control, and enough balance between all these considerations to live a healthy and happy life.

For references on hormones and diet control, here is a list that should help you with hormones, the why, how, and what they do:

http://www.bodybuilding.com/fun/6-easy-steps-to-ensuring-hormones-keep-you-lean.html

http://www.pennmedicine.org/health_info/body_guide/reftext/html/endo_sys_fin.html

http://en.wikipedia.org/wiki/Endocrine_gland

http://www.food-first-wellness.com/basic-hormones.html

Copy any one of the listed references and paste them on your URL (address bar on the top of your page).

# Factors Affecting Metabolic Demands

As you progress in your workouts, you should consider "density" as one of the variables.
Density of training is the amount of work performed during your workout period. It's important because it affects what the body does with its hormones.
Usually the intensity of the exercise is ever increasing as a trainee progresses in his workout routine.
Muscle tissue requires stimulation and it gets it by increasing the work load.
Let's look at how density can be utilized.

If you increase the tension duration per set time, as in slowing down the time of each repetition while keeping the same weight (load), you must also reduce the rest interval.
As an example of how this works is if the time duration increases by 8 seconds, you'll have to decrease the rest interval by 8 seconds.

If you increase the repetition number for the per set time, you will have to increase the speed of each rep or decrease the rest interval between sets.

If you increase the load (resistance or weight used) per set time in doing the same number of reps, you will then increase the density for that period of time.

If you use the same load and decrease the time, you'll increase the density.

The reason density is so important is that as it increases in your workouts, it also places a greater demand on your metabolism. When density increases, catabolic changes occur in the muscles. The muscle fibers have taken stress, and need time to heal (anabolic changes). This occurs during rest and especially during sleep, as in the 3$^{rd}$ and 4$^{th}$ stages of REM sleep. The result is in body composition adaptations such as increased strength, decreased body fat and increased levels of testosterone and growth (GH) hormone production.

GH is released from the anterior pituitary gland and it stimulates the secretion of a family of insulin-like growth factor (IGF) hormones. These, along with GH, stimulate skeletal growth in children.

GH does its work in stimulating protein synthesis in many tissues, increases fat oxidation (fat burning), elevates the release of fatty acids from fat tissues, and boosts resting caloric expenditure (i.e. basal metabolic rate). Another function of GH is that it inhibits the uptake of glucose by the muscle tissue while stimulating uptake of amino acids. The amino acids are used in the synthesis of proteins, and the muscle shifts to using fatty acids as a source of energy.

As one ages, there is a decline in GH secretion and this also occurs in people with histories of traumatic brain injury (any head injury that caused a loss of consciousness), sleep problems, and in chronic illness. In contact sports, with repetitive head trauma, there is often a dysfunction of an area of the brain called the hypothalamus. This area of the brain controls the regulation of many hormones, including GH.

GH therapy in GH deficient patients decreases body fat and increases muscle mass, bone density, and energy levels. Too much GH can cause joint swelling, joint pain, carpal tunnel syndrome, an increased risk of diabetes, and decreased thyroid functions have been reported.

There is a growth hormone releasing hormone (GHRH) used by some doctors to stimulate the pituitary release of GH.

Suggestion: Let the body regulate its need of hormonal levels by itself, unless there are specific reasons for outside sources to assist in curing an abnormality.

# References

## Exercise

1. Rodriquez NR, Di Marco NM, Langley S (2009) American College of Sports Medicine position stand. Nutrition and athletic performance. Med Sci sports Exerc 41
2. Malina RM (2007) Body composition in athletes: assessment and estimated fatness. Clin Sports Med 26: 37-68.doi: 10.1016/j.csm.2006.11.004
3. Nattiv A, Loucks AB, Manore MM, Sanborn CF, Sindgot-Borgen J, et a; / (2007) American College pf Sports Medicine position stand. The female athlete triad. Med Sic Sports Exec 39: 1867-1882.
4. Alva B, Winner R, and Dodd DJ (2010). The effect of daily undulated per- iodization as compared to linear periodization in strength gains of collegiate athletes, Journal of Strength and Conditioning Research, 24 (suppl. 1), 1.
5. Berry M, and Ebben B. (2001),. Free weight variable resistance. In Strength Cats. Retrieved from http://strengthcats.Com/variableresistance.htm
6. American College of Sports Medicine (ACSM).
7. No Gym Needed – Quick & Simple Workouts for Busy Guys: Get a 'Fit' Body in 30 Minutes or Less! By Lise Cartwright (Kindle Edition)
8. Exercise Physiology: Theory and Application to Fitness and Performance. By Scott Powers (Hardcover).

9. DeFranco J (2004) Football conditioning: The right way! In DeFranco's Training. Retrieved from http://www.defrancostrainning.com/ask-joe.html?start+16.
10. Buchenholz DH (2004) The best sports training book ever! N.l.: Inno-Sport.
11. Fleck JP, and Kraemer WJ ((1987) Designing resistance training programs. Champaign, IL: Human Kinetics.
12. Strength Training by the National Strength & Conditioning Association, Lee E. Brown, Editor, Copyright (2007) by NSCA.
13. NASM Essentials of Personal Fitness Training, 3rd Edition, Clark MA, Lucett SC, Corn RJ, Editors.
14. Burd NA,low-load high volume resistance exercise stimulates muscle protein
   Synthesis more than high-load low volume resistance exercise in young men.
   PLoS One, 2010 Aug 9;5(8):e 12033.

# Diet

1. American Chemical Society. "Sustainable Farm Practices Improve Third World Food Production" (press release, January 23, 2006).
2. International Food Information Council. "2008 Food & Health Survey: Consumer Attitudes toward Food, Nutrition, and Health. May 14, 2008 Council. http://www.ific.org.
3. Rosenbaum M, and RL Leibel. 2010. Adaptive thermogenesis in humans. Int J
   Obes (Lond). 34 (SUppl 1):S47-S55

4. Barr SI, 2003 Increased dairy product or calcium intake: Is body weight or

Composition affected in humans? J Nutr. 133(1):245S-248S.

5. Feskanich D, et.al. 1997. Milk, Dietary calcium, and bone fractures in women; A
12-year prospective study. Am J Public Health. 87(6):992-97.

6. Kessler DA 2009. The End of Overeating: Taking Control of the Insatiable
American Appetite. New York: Rodale.

## Sleep

1. Becker PM. "Insomnia: Prevalence, Impact, Pathogenesis, Differential Diagnosis,
And Evaluation," Psychiatric Clinics of North America (Dec. 2006): Col. 29, No. 4,
pp.855-70.

2. Meltzer TA, "Sleep and Anxiety Disorders," Psychiatric Clinics of North America
(Dec. 2006): Vol. 29, No. 4, pp.1059-.

3. National Institute of Neurological Disorders and Stroke. "Brain Basics:
Understanding Sleep," fact sheet updated May 21, 2007.

4. Walker MP. "The Role of Sleep in Cognition and Emotion," Annals of the New
York Academy of Sciences (March 2009): Vol. 1156, pp. 168-.

5. Epstein L, ed., Improving Sleep, Harvard Medical School Special Health Report,
2008.

6. Harvey AG. "Sleep and Circadian Rhythms in Bipolar Disorder: Seeking
Synchrony, Harmony, and Regulation," American Journal of Psychiatry (July
2008): Vol.165, No. 7. Pp820-.

7. ScienceDaily – Free subscription on sleep/other subjects – excellent.

http://feedburner.google.com/fb/a/mailverify?uri=scien cedaily/most_popular

# Hormones

1. Hormonal Balance, How to lose Weight by Understanding Your Hormones and Metabolism by Scott Isaacs MD, FACP, FACE: 3$^{rd}$ Edition.
2. Church TS., et al. Trends over 5 Decades in U.S. Occupation-Related Physical Activity and Their Associations with Obesity. PLoS One, 2011;6(5);e19657
3. Carhuatanta KA, et al. Voluntary Exercise Improves High-Fat Diet-Induced Leptin Resistance Independent of Adiposity. Endocrinology. 2011; Jul; 152(7):2655-2664.
4. Folland JP, Williams AG. The Adaptations to Strength Training: Morphological and Neurological Contributions to Increased Strength. Sports Medicine. 2007; 37(2):145-168.
5. Gabriel DA, Kamen G, Frost G. Neural Adaptations to Resistance Exercise: Mechanisms and Recommendation for Training Practices, Sports Medicine. 2006;36(2):133-149.
6. Hotchkiss AK, et al. Fifteen Years after "Wingspread": Environmental Endocrine Disrupters and Human and Wildlife Health: Where We Are Today and Where We

Need to Go. Toxicology and Chemistry. 2004 Aug;23(8): 1928-1938.

7.    Knutson KL, Van Cauter E. Associations between Sleep Loss and Increased
Risk of Obesity and Diabeter.   Annals of the New York Academy of Sciences.
2008; 1129:287-304.